OSTEOPOROSIS DIET COOKBOOK 2024

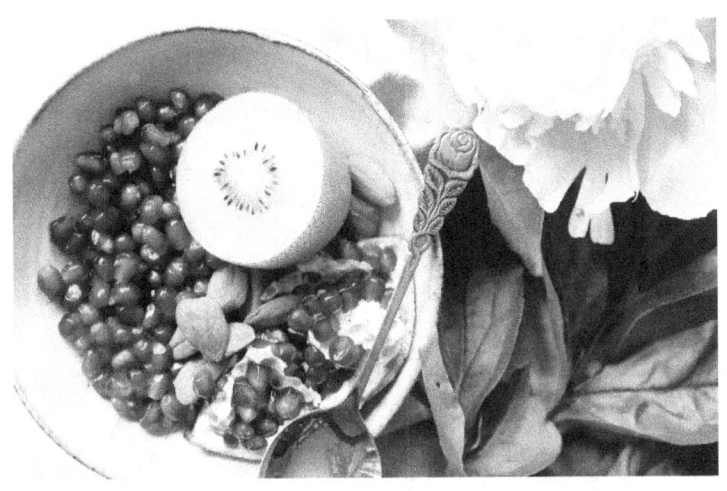

Nutritional Recipes for Stronger Bones and Better Health

Misty J. Font

Copyright © Misty J. Font 2023

All rights reserved. No part of this publication may be reproduced, distributed, or transmitted in any form or by any means, including photocopying, recording, or other electronic or mechanical methods, without the prior written permission of the publisher, except in the case of brief quotations embodied in critical reviews and certain other noncommercial uses permitted by copyright law.

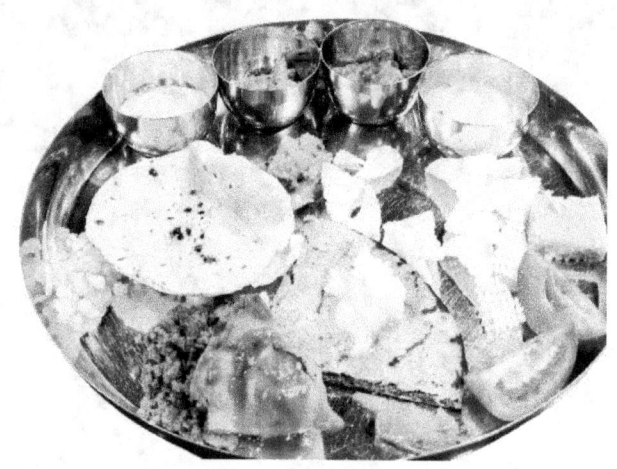

Table of content

CHAPTER 1: INTRODUCTION...7
   Understanding Osteoporosis............................... 11
CHAPTER 2: OSTEOPOROSIS BASICS.................13
   What is osteoporosis... 13
   Risk factors for osteoporosis................................ 14
   Symptoms and diagnoses.................................... 14
CHAPTER 3: BREAKFAST RECIPES....................... 16
   Spinach and feta omelet....................................... 16
   Greek Yogurt Parfait... 17
   Whole-Grain Pancakes..18
   Avocado toast with poached eggs...................... 19
   Berry Smoothie... 19
   Quinoa Breakfast Bowl... 20
   Chia Seed Pudding..21
   Egg and Vegetable Breakfast Burrito...................22
   Steel cut oatmeal with almonds and berries...........22
   Salmon & Cream Cheese Bagel...........................23
   Cottage Cheese With Pineapple..........................24
   Mushroom and Spinach frittata............................25
   Banana Walnut Muffins...26
   Veggie and cheese breakfast quesadilla............. 27
   Peanut Butter and Banana Toast.........................28
CHAPTER 4: LUNCHTIME RECIPES........................ 29
   Grilled Salmon Salad.. 29
   Quinoa & Black Bean Bowl...................................30
   Chicken and Vegetable Stir-Fry........................... 31
   Spinach and Feta Stuffed Chicken Breasts........... 32

Mediterranean Chickpea Salad............... 33
Turkey and Avocado Wrap...................... 33
Vegetarian Lentil Soup..............................34
Tuna Salad, Lettuce Wraps........................ 35
Veggie and Quinoa Stuffed Bell Peppers............... 36
Greek Chicken Salad.......................................37
Salmon and asparagus quiche........................... 38
Caprese Salad... 39
Turkey and Spinach Wrap............................. 40
Eggplant and Tomato Panini.......................41
Vegetable and Tofu Stir-fry.......................... 42

CHAPTER 5: DINNER RECIPES..........................44
Baked Salmon with Lemon and Dill............... 44
Vegetable and Chickpea Curry............................ 45
Grilled Chicken and Vegetable Skewers................46
Mushroom with Spinach Stuffed Chicken Breasts.. 47
Vegetarian Lentil Shepherd's Pie.........................48
Salmon and Asparagus Sheet Pan Dinner............ 50
Turkey and Vegetable Stir-Fry............................. 51
Vegetable and Tofu Stir Fry with Brown Rice..........52
Baked Eggplant Parmesan.................................. 53
Stuffed bell peppers with quinoa and black beans. 55
Lemon Garlic Shrimp Pasta.................................. 56
Vegetable and Tofu Noodle Stir-Fry........................ 57
Baked Chicken Parmesan..................................... 59
Vegetarian Spinach and Mushroom Lasagna..........60
Vegetable and Lentil Curry.................................... 62

CHAPTER 6: SNACK AND SIDE DISH RECIPES......64

Greek Yogurt and Mixed Berries..................64
Cottage Cheese and Pineapple Skewers..............64
Hummus and Vegetable Platter....................65
Trail mix with nuts and seeds...................65
Whole Grain Crackers with Avocado Mash........... 66
Steamed broccoli with garlic butter....................67
Quinoa Salad With Cranberries and Almonds........ 67
Roasted Brussels sprouts with Balsamic Glaze..... 68
Caprese Salad Skewers................................. 69
Sweet Potato Fries.................................... 70
Mango salsa... 71
Zucchini Noodles With Pesto..........................71
Cucumber and Tomato Salad............................ 72
Edamame Hummus.......................................73
Stuffed bell peppers with quinoa and vegetables... 74

CHAPTER 7: DESSERTS AND SWEET TREATS...... 76
Greek yogurt parfait with fresh fruit..............76
Baked apples with cinnamon......................... 77
Dark chocolate-dipped strawberries................. 78
Frozen Banana Pops................................. 78
Chia Seed Pudding...................................79
Frozen Yogurt Bark................................. 80
Baked peaches with cinnamon and honey............ 81
Coconut Date Balls................................. 82
Homemade Fruit Sorbet.............................. 83
Pumpkin Oatmeal Cookies............................ 84

CHAPTER 8 : BEVERAGES..............................86
Calcium-Rich Smoothie.............................. 86

Almond Milk...87
Green Tea..88
Bone-building Berry Smoothie..............................88
Calcium-boosting Orange Smoothie.....................89
Strawberry Kiwi Calcium Smoothie.......................90
Homemade Cashew Milk...91
Banana-Almond Smoothie......................................92
Vanilla almond milk..92
Chocolate almond milk... 93
Golden milk (turmeric latte)...................................94

CHAPTER 9: BONUSES 7-DAY MEAL PLANNING...96
CONCLUSION...101
Additional materials... 101

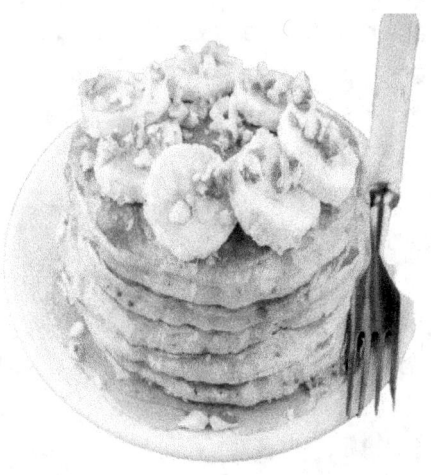

CHAPTER 1: INTRODUCTION

Once upon a time, in a lovely little village nestled amidst rolling hills and lush vegetation, Merry, a vivacious and joyful woman who exuded warmth wherever she went. Merry was known for her enormous energy and zest for life, but she had no idea that her journey would take an unexpected turn.

Merry stumbled and fell one sunny afternoon while gardening in her backyard, sending a stinging ache through her wrist as she sought to brace herself. She dismissed the occurrence as a small error and went about her regular routine, but the pain in her wrist persisted, steadily worsening over time. Concerned, Merry went to the doctor, only to learn that she had osteoporosis, a condition characterized by weakening bones that are prone to fractures.

Merry, shocked and dismayed by the news, faced a tough challenge. As someone who valued her active lifestyle, the prospect of being constrained by brittle bones filled her with anxiety. Determined to take control of her health, Merry went on a journey for information, looking for resources to help her manage the challenges of managing osteoporosis.

During her quest, Merry discovered a valuable resource: the Osteoporosis Diet Cookbook. Merry enthusiastically plunged into its pages, devouring every word with intense determination, piqued by the promise of replenishing her body with bone-boosting nutrients.

Merry was enthralled by the abundance of information in the cookbook as she flipped through it. From grasping the significance of calcium-rich foods to finding the power of vitamin D in bone health, each page provided essential insights on designing a diet to promote her recovery.

Merry, armed with fresh information and a revitalized sense of purpose, set out on a culinary expedition, transforming her kitchen into a healing laboratory. With the Osteoporosis Diet Cookbook as her guide, she began on a journey of discovery, experimenting with a variety of clean foods to create tasty and nutritious meals that would nourish her body from within.

From vivid salads bursting with fresh greens and crunchy nuts to hearty soups full with healthful grains and lean proteins, Merry embraced the art of cooking wholeheartedly, infusing each dish with love and intention. With each bite, she savored the flavors of healing, knowing that each ingredient was an important component in her quest to strengthen her bones and restore her vitality.

As the weeks progressed into months, Merry's hard work began to pay off, literally. With each passing day, she felt her strength returning, her bones becoming stronger with each nutritious meal. The days of uncertainty and dread had passed, giving way to a profound sense of resilience and empowerment.

Merry's success inspired her to share her experience with others, spreading the message of hope and healing far and wide. She motivated countless people to see the importance of diet in healing their bodies and restoring their health.

Today, when Merry tends to her garden once more, she does so with a renewed sense of appreciation and vibrancy, her spirit as alive as the petals around her. Merry continues to relish each day with the Osteoporosis Diet Cookbook by her side, knowing that her journey to recovery is a tribute to the human spirit's perseverance and the transformative power of nutrition.

Understanding Osteoporosis

Osteoporosis, also known as the "silent disease," causes weakening bones that are prone to fractures. It affects millions of people globally, primarily postmenopausal women and elderly adults. Understanding the underlying causes of osteoporosis is critical for taking preventive efforts to reduce its impact on your health.

Nutrition is essential for maintaining bone health and managing osteoporosis. Adequate intake of vital nutrients like calcium, vitamin D, vitamin K, magnesium, and phosphorus is critical for maintaining bone density and strength. Conversely, deficits in these nutrients can hasten bone loss and raise the risk of fracture. You can maximize your nutritional intake by making smart dietary choices and using strategic supplementation to maintain bone health and slow the course of osteoporosis.

This cookbook is a comprehensive resource for preparing delicious and nutritious meals that promote bone health and help osteoporosis management. It allows you to take control of your diet and make informed decisions that prioritize your bone health by providing nutrient-dense recipes, practical meal plans, and evidence-based nutritional recommendations.

Whether you want to avoid osteoporosis, control its progression, or just follow a bone-friendly diet as part of a healthy lifestyle, this cookbook provides a wealth of culinary inspiration and practical ideas to help you get stronger, healthier bones.

CHAPTER 2: OSTEOPOROSIS BASICS

Welcome to Part 2 of the Osteoporosis Diet Cookbook, where we'll look at the fundamentals of osteoporosis, from description to diagnosis. Understanding the foundations of osteoporosis is essential for taking proactive efforts to manage and reduce its effects on your health.

What is osteoporosis

Osteoporosis is a chronic illness in which bones deteriorate, making them more fragile and prone to fracture. Osteoporosis, also known as the "silent disease," can progress quietly, with no obvious signs until a fracture occurs. Bone is a dynamic substance that is constantly remodeling, but osteoporosis disrupts the balance between bone creation and bone resorption, resulting in a net decrease of bone density over time.

Risk factors for osteoporosis

Numerous variables contribute to the development of osteoporosis, some of which are changeable and others that are inherent in individual traits. Age, gender, and heredity all play important roles, with postmenopausal women and older adults being at a higher risk. Sedentary behavior, smoking, excessive alcohol intake, and poor nutrition are all risk factors for bone loss. Additionally, certain medical conditions and drugs can raise the risk of developing osteoporosis.

Symptoms and diagnoses

Osteoporosis may not cause symptoms in its early stages, making detection difficult without thorough monitoring. However, as the condition advances, people may have symptoms including back discomfort, loss of height, and fractures, notably in the spine, hip, or wrist. Clinical examination, imaging techniques such as bone density scans (DEXA), and laboratory testing to determine bone turnover markers are commonly used in the diagnosis.

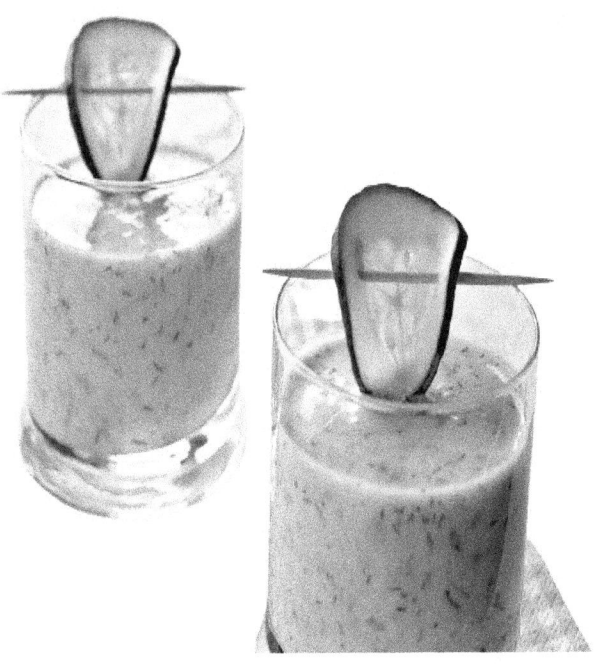

CHAPTER 3: BREAKFAST RECIPES

Spinach and feta omelet

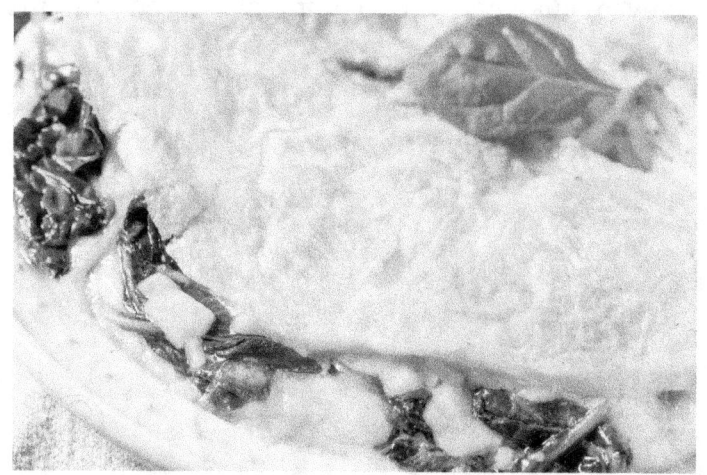

Ingredients:

- Eggs.
- Fresh spinach.
- Feta cheese
- Olive oil

Instructions:
1. In a medium-size skillet, heat the olive oil.
2. Sauté the spinach until wilted.
3. Beat the eggs and pour them into the skillet.
4. Sprinkle crumbled feta cheese over the eggs.
5. Cook until the omelette has set and turned golden brown.

Greek Yogurt Parfait

Ingredients:
- Greek Yogurt.
- Fresh berries (blueberries, strawberries, and raspberries)
- Granola
- Honey (Optional)

Instructions:
- In a glass or dish, combine Greek yogurt, berries, and granola.
- Drizzle with honey if preferred.

- Serve cold.

Whole-Grain Pancakes

Ingredients:
- Whole wheat flour.
- Baking Powder
- Milk (plant-based milk)
- Eggs
- Vanilla extract.

Instructions:
1. In a bowl, combine the whole wheat flour and baking powder.
2. Add the milk, eggs, and vanilla essence to the dry ingredients and stir until combined.
3. To create pancakes, heat a skillet over medium heat and pour the batter in.
4. Cook until bubbles appear on the surface, then flip and finish till golden brown.

Avocado toast with poached eggs

Ingredients:
- whole grain bread.
- Ripe avocado and eggs.
- Salt and pepper.

Instructions:
1. Toast the whole grain bread till golden brown.
2. Season the toast with salt and pepper, then mash in the ripe avocado.
3. Poach an egg and serve on top of the avocado toast.
4. If needed, season with extra salt and pepper.

Berry Smoothie

Ingredients:
- mixed berries (strawberries, blueberries, raspberries).

- Spinach Greek yogurt
- Almond milk (or other milk)
- Honey (Optional)

Instructions:

1. Blend together the berries, spinach, Greek yogurt, almond milk, and honey until smooth.
2. If desired, add extra honey to adjust the sweetness.
3. Serve cold.

Quinoa Breakfast Bowl

Ingredients:

- Cooked Quinoa.
- Almond milk (or other milk)
- Chopped nuts (almonds and walnuts)
- Sliced banana
- Cinnamon

Instructions:

1. In a bowl, combine cooked quinoa and almond milk.
2. Finish with chopped nuts, sliced banana, and a sprinkle of cinnamon.
3. Stir until combined and serve warm.

Chia Seed Pudding

Ingredients:
1. chia seeds.
2. Almond milk (or other milk)
3. Add vanilla extract and honey (optional).
4. Serve with sliced strawberries and kiwi.
5. Combine the chia seeds, almond milk, vanilla essence, and honey in a bowl.
6. Refrigerate for at least 2 hours or overnight to thicken.
7. Serve topped with sliced fruit.

Egg and Vegetable Breakfast Burrito

Ingredients:
- whole grain tortilla.
- Ingredients: eggs, diced bell peppers (of any color), onion, and spinach.
- Shredded cheese (optional).

Instructions:
1. In a skillet, scramble the eggs until cooked through.
2. Cook the diced bell peppers, onion, and spinach in the skillet until soft.
3. Warm the tortilla, then fill it with the scrambled egg mixture.
4. If desired, sprinkle with shredded cheese before rolling it into a tortilla.

Steel cut oatmeal with almonds and berries

Ingredients:
- Steel cut oats.
- Ingredients: water and sliced almonds.
- Mixed Berries
- Maple syrup (optional).

Instructions:
1. Cook the steel cut oats according to the package instructions.
2. Serve with sliced almonds, mixed berries, and a drizzle of maple syrup, if desired.

Salmon & Cream Cheese Bagel

Ingredients:
- Whole grain bagels.
- Smoked salmon
- Cream Cheese

- Sliced cucumber
- Fresh dill.

Instructions:
1. Toast the whole-grain bagel until golden brown.
2. Spread cream cheese over the bagel halves.
3. Garnish with smoked salmon, sliced cucumber, and fresh dill.

Cottage Cheese With Pineapple

Ingredients:
- cottage cheese.
- Fresh pineapple chunks.
- Chopped nuts (pecans and almonds)
- Honey (Optional)

Instructions:
1. Serve the cottage cheese in a bowl.

2. Garnish with fresh pineapple pieces and chopped nuts.
3. Drizzle with honey if preferred.

Mushroom and Spinach frittata

Ingredients:
- Eggs.
- Fresh spinach, sliced mushrooms, and diced onion.
- Olive oil

Instructions:
1. Preheat the oven to 350°F (175°C).
2. Sauté the mushrooms and onion in olive oil until soft.
3. Beat eggs and pour into a greased baking dish.
4. Add the sautéed mushrooms and spinach to the eggs.

5. Bake for 20-25 minutes, or until the frittata has set.

Banana Walnut Muffins

Ingredients:
- whole wheat flour.
- Baking Powder
- Ripe bananas.
- Chopped walnuts.
- Greek yogurt
- Honey

Instructions:
1. Preheat the oven to 350°F/175°C and line a muffin tray with liners.
2. In a bowl, combine the whole wheat flour and baking powder.
3. Mash ripe bananas and combine in Greek yogurt and honey.

4. Combine wet and dry ingredients, then fold in the chopped walnuts.
5. Place the batter in the muffin tin and bake for 20-25 minutes.

Veggie and cheese breakfast quesadilla

Ingredients:
- whole grain tortilla.
- Scrambled eggs.
- Diced bell peppers, any hue.
- Diced tomatoes.
- Shredded cheese

Instructions:
1. Heat the whole grain tortilla in a skillet.
2. Spread scrambled eggs, diced bell peppers, diced tomatoes, and shredded cheese on one half of the tortilla.

3. Fold the tortilla in half and cook until the cheese melts and the quesadilla turns golden brown.

Peanut Butter and Banana Toast

Ingredients:
- whole grain bread.
- Peanut Butter
- Sliced banana
- Chia seeds (optional).

Instructions:
1. Toast the whole grain bread till golden brown.
2. Spread peanut butter on bread.
3. Top with sliced banana and chia seeds, if preferred.

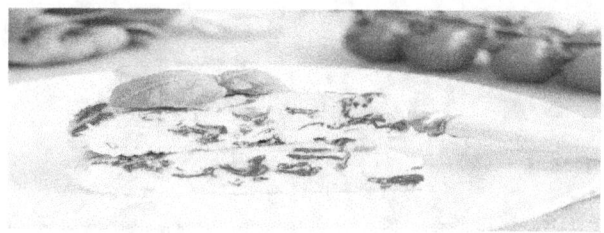

CHAPTER 4: LUNCHTIME RECIPES

Grilled Salmon Salad

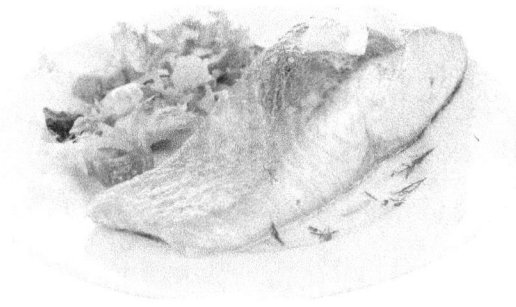

Ingredients:

- Salmon filet
- Mixed greens (spinach, arugula, and kale).
- Cherry tomatoes
- Cucumber (sliced) with olive oil
- Lemon juice

Instructions:

1. Grill the salmon fillet until cooked through.
2. Toss the mixed greens, cherry tomatoes, and cucumber with olive oil and lemon juice.
3. Add grilled fish to the salad.

Quinoa & Black Bean Bowl

Ingredients:

- Cooked Quinoa.
- Black beans
- Avocado, diced
- Diced red bell pepper with lime juice.
- cilantro, chopped

Instructions:

- Combine cooked quinoa and black beans in a bowl.
- Include diced avocado and red bell pepper.

- Drizzle with lime juice and garnish with chopped cilantro.

Chicken and Vegetable Stir-Fry

Ingredients:
- Sliced chicken breast.
- broccoli florets
- Sliced bell peppers (any color) with julienned carrots
- Soy sauce
- garlic, minced
- Ginger, grated

Instructions:
1. Cook the chicken breast slices in a skillet.
2. Add the broccoli florets, bell peppers, and carrots to the skillet.
3. Add soy sauce, minced garlic, and grated ginger.
4. Cook until vegetables are soft and crunchy.

Spinach and Feta Stuffed Chicken Breasts

Ingredients:

- Chicken breast
- Fresh spinach leaves.
- Feta cheese
- Garlic powder
- Olive oil

Instructions:

1. Preheat the oven to 375° Fahrenheit (190° Celsius).
2. Butterfly the chicken breast and load it with fresh spinach and crumbled feta cheese.
3. Season with garlic powder and drizzle with olive oil.
4. Bake for 25-30 minutes, or until the chicken is cooked through.

Mediterranean Chickpea Salad

Ingredients:
1. cooked chickpeas, chopped cucumber, split cherry tomatoes, pitted Kalamata olives, thinly sliced red onion, crumbled feta cheese, and olive oil.
2. Red wine vinegar
3. Fresh oregano, chopped.
4. Mix chickpeas, cucumber, cherry tomatoes, Kalamata olives, red onion, and feta cheese in a bowl.
5. Dress with olive oil, red wine vinegar, and freshly chopped oregano.
6. Toss gently to mix before serving cold.

Turkey and Avocado Wrap

Ingredients:
- whole grain tortilla.
- Sliced Turkey Breast

- Avocado mashed with lettuce leaves.
- Sliced tomato with Dijon mustard (optional).

Instructions:
1. Lay down the whole-grain tortilla.
2. Spread mashed avocado on the tortilla.
3. Layer the sliced turkey breast, lettuce leaves, and tomato slices.
4. If preferred, add a dollop of Dijon mustard.
5. Roll the tortilla tightly and cut into halves.

Vegetarian Lentil Soup

Ingredients:
- Lentils.
- Diced carrots, celery, onion, and minced garlic
- Vegetable broth with bay leaves.
- Italian seasoning.

Instructions:

1. Cook diced carrots, celery, onion, and minced garlic in a saucepan until softened.
2. Combine the lentils, vegetable broth, bay leaves, and Italian spice.
3. Bring to a boil, then reduce the heat and simmer until the lentils are cooked.
4. Remove the bay leaves before serving.

Tuna Salad, Lettuce Wraps

Ingredients:
- drained canned tuna with Greek yogurt.
- Celery, diced
- Red onions, diced
- Dill pickles, diced
- lettuce leaves

Instructions:
1. Combine canned tuna, Greek yogurt, diced celery, red onion, and dill pickle in a mixing dish.

2. Spoon the tuna salad onto the lettuce leaves.
3. Roll up the lettuce leaves into wraps.

Veggie and Quinoa Stuffed Bell Peppers

Ingredients:
- Bell peppers.
- Cooked quinoa and sliced zucchini.
- Diced yellow squash with tomato sauce.
- Italian seasoning.
- Shredded cheese (optional).

Instructions:
1. Preheat the oven to 375° Fahrenheit (190° Celsius).
2. Cut the tops of bell peppers and remove the seeds.
3. In a bowl, combine cooked quinoa, diced zucchini, yellow squash, tomato sauce, and Italian seasoning.

4. Stuff the bell peppers with the quinoa and vegetable combination.
5. Sprinkle with shredded cheese if desired.
6. Bake for 25–30 minutes, or until the peppers are soft.

Greek Chicken Salad

Ingredients:

- Grilled chicken breast, diced Romaine lettuce, chopped
- Cucumber, diced
- Cherry tomatoes, halved
- Kalamata olives, pitted
- Red onion, thinly sliced
- Feta cheese, crumbled
- Greek vinaigrette dressing

Instructions:

1. together grilled chicken breast, romaine lettuce, cucumber, cherry tomatoes, Kalamata olives, red onion, and feta cheese in a bowl.
2. Drizzle with Greek vinaigrette and toss to coat.
3. Serve cold.

Salmon and asparagus quiche

Ingredients:
- Pie crust.
- Salmon fillet, cooked, flakes
- asparagus spears, blanched and cut
- Eggs
- Milk (or Cream)
- Shredded cheese
- Salt and pepper.

Instructions:
1. Preheat the oven to 375° Fahrenheit (190° Celsius).

2. Line a pie plate with pie crust.
3. Spread cooked, flaked salmon and chopped asparagus over the pie crust.
4. In a mixing dish, combine eggs, milk, shredded cheese, salt, and pepper.
5. Pour egg mixture over fish and asparagus.
6. Bake for 35-40 minutes, or until the quiche is firm and golden brown.

Caprese Salad

Ingredients:

- Fresh mozzarella cheese
- Sliced tomato
- Fresh basil leaves.
- Balsamic glaze
- Olive oil
- Salt and pepper.

Instructions:

1. Place alternate pieces of fresh mozzarella cheese and tomato on a platter.
2. Tuck fresh basil leaves between the tomato and cheese slices.
3. Drizzle with the balsamic glaze and olive oil.
4. Season with salt and pepper to taste.

Turkey and Spinach Wrap

Ingredients:
- whole grain tortilla.
- Sliced Turkey Breast
- Fresh spinach leaves.
- Hummus
- roasted red peppers, sliced

Instructions:
1. Spread hummus over a whole grain tortilla.
2. Layer sliced turkey breast with fresh spinach leaves and roasted red peppers.
3. Roll the tortilla tightly and cut into halves.

Eggplant and Tomato Panini

Ingredients:

- whole grain bread.
- Eggplant chopped and grilled
- Tomato sliced
- Fresh basil leaves.
- Mozzarella cheese, sliced
- Olive oil
- Balsamic glaze

Instructions:

1. Preheat the panini press or grill pan.
2. Place grilled eggplant slices, tomato slices, fresh basil leaves, and mozzarella cheese between slices of whole grain bread.
3. Drizzle olive oil on the outside of the bread slices.
4. Grill the panini until the bread is golden brown and the cheese melts.

5. Drizzle with balsamic glaze before serving.

Vegetable and Tofu Stir-fry

Ingredients:
- Cubed firm tofu and broccoli florets.
- Snap peas
- sliced carrots, bell peppers (any color), and soy sauce.
- Sesame oil
- garlic, minced
- Ginger, grated

Instructions:
1. Stir-fry the cubed tofu in sesame oil until golden brown.
2. Add the broccoli florets, snap peas, sliced carrots, and sliced bell peppers to the skillet.
3. Stir in the minced garlic and grated ginger.
4. Drizzle with soy sauce and heat until the vegetables are soft and crispy.

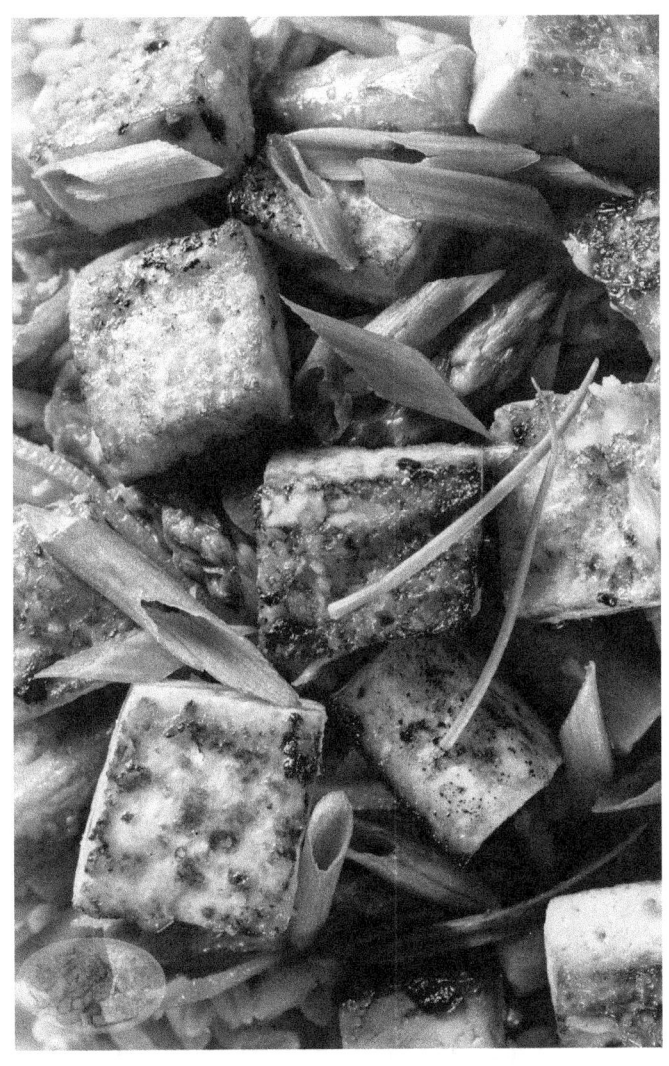

CHAPTER 5: DINNER RECIPES

Baked Salmon with Lemon and Dill

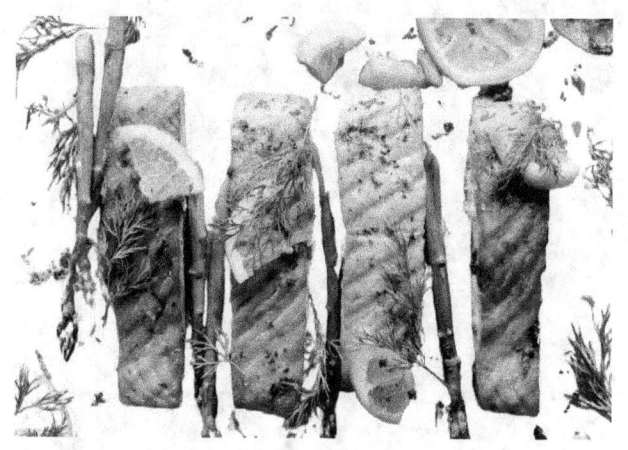

Ingredients:

- Salmon fillets
- Lemon slices
- Fresh dill.
- Olive oil
- Salt and pepper.

Instructions:
1. Preheat the oven to 375° Fahrenheit (190° Celsius).
2. Place the salmon fillets on a parchment-lined baking sheet.
3. Drizzle with olive oil, then season with salt and pepper.
4. Garnish with lemon slices and fresh dill.
5. Bake the salmon for 12-15 minutes, or until thoroughly done.

Vegetable and Chickpea Curry

Ingredients:
- Cooked chickpeas.
- Mixed vegetables (including bell peppers, carrots, and cauliflower)
- Coconut milk
- Curry paste
- Onions, diced
- garlic, minced

- Ginger, grated
- Olive oil

Instructions:

1. In a large pot or skillet, heat the olive oil.
2. Sauté the diced onion, minced garlic, and grated ginger until fragrant.
3. Add the mixed vegetables and cooked chickpeas to the skillet.
4. Stir in the coconut milk and curry paste.
5. Simmer for 15-20 minutes, until the vegetables are soft.

Grilled Chicken and Vegetable Skewers

Ingredients:

- cubed chicken breast, diced bell peppers (any color), diced red onion, sliced zucchini, and cherry tomatoes.
- Olive oil with Italian spice.
- Salt and pepper.

Instructions:
1. Preheat the grill to medium-high heat.
2. Thread chicken chunks and chopped vegetables onto skewers.
3. Drizzle with olive oil and season with Italian seasoning, salt, and pepper.
4. Grill the skewers for 10-12 minutes, flipping regularly, until the chicken is fully cooked and the veggies are soft.

Mushroom with Spinach Stuffed Chicken Breasts

Ingredients:
- chicken breast.
- mushrooms, sliced
- Fresh spinach leaves.
- garlic, minced
- Olive oil

- Shredded mozzarella cheese.
- Salt and pepper.

Instructions:

1. Preheat the oven to 375° Fahrenheit (190° Celsius).
2. In a medium-size skillet, heat the olive oil.
3. Sauté sliced mushrooms and minced garlic until they are soft.
4. Butterfly chicken breast and stuff with sautéed mushrooms and fresh spinach leaves.
5. Sprinkle with shredded mozzarella cheese and season with salt and pepper.
6. Bake for 25-30 minutes, or until the chicken is cooked through.

Vegetarian Lentil Shepherd's Pie

Ingredients:
- Cooked lentils.

- Mixed vegetables (including carrots, peas, and corn)
- Dice the onion and mince the garlic.
- Vegetable broth
- Tomato paste
- Mashed potatoes
- Olive oil

Instructions:

1. Preheat the oven to 375° Fahrenheit (190° Celsius).
2. Cook diced onion and minced garlic in olive oil until tender.
3. Add the cooked lentils, mixed veggies, vegetable broth, and tomato paste to the skillet.
4. Simmer for 10-15 minutes, until the mixture thickens.
5. Place the lentil mixture in a baking dish and top with mashed potatoes.

6. Bake for 25-30 minutes, or until the mashed potatoes turn golden brown.

Salmon and Asparagus Sheet Pan Dinner

Ingredients:
- salmon fillets.
- asparagus spears
- Cherry tomatoes
- Lemon slices
- Ingredients include olive oil and garlic powder.
- Salt and pepper.

Instructions:
1. Preheat the oven to 400° F (200° C).
2. Place salmon fillets, asparagus spears, and cherry tomatoes on a parchment-lined baking sheet.

3. Drizzle olive oil and season with garlic powder, salt, and pepper.
4. Top the salmon with lemon wedges.
5. Bake for 12-15 minutes, or until the fish and veggies are soft.

Turkey and Vegetable Stir-Fry

Ingredients:
- Ground turkey.
- Mixed vegetables (including bell peppers, broccoli, and snap peas)
- Onions, diced
- garlic, minced
- Ginger, grated
- Soy sauce
- Sesame oil
- Olive oil

Instructions:

1. Heat the olive oil in a big skillet or wok over high heat.
2. Cook the ground turkey until browned.
3. Stir in the diced onion, minced garlic, and grated ginger.
4. Stir-fry the mixed vegetables in the skillet until they are soft and crispy.
5. Toss with soy sauce and sesame oil until well combined.

Vegetable and Tofu Stir Fry with Brown Rice

Ingredients:
- Cubed firm tofu.
- Mixed vegetables (including broccoli, bell peppers, and carrots)
- Ingredients: chopped onion, minced garlic, grated ginger.
- Soy sauce

- Sesame oil
- Brown rice, cooked.

Instructions:
1. Heat the sesame oil in a big skillet or wok over high heat.
2. Add the cubed tofu and heat until golden brown.
3. Stir in the sliced onion, minced garlic, and grated ginger.
4. Stir-fry the mixed vegetables in the skillet until they are soft and crispy.
5. Drizzle with soy sauce and mix well.
6. Serve with cooked brown rice.

Baked Eggplant Parmesan

Ingredients:
- Sliced eggplant and Marinara sauce.
- Shredded mozzarella cheese.
- Grated Parmesan cheese.

- Italian breadcrumbs
- Season with olive oil, salt, and pepper.

Instructions:

1. Preheat the oven to 375° Fahrenheit (190° Celsius).
2. Dip eggplant slices in beaten egg and cover with Italian breadcrumbs.
3. Place the breaded eggplant slices on a baking sheet with parchment paper.
4. Drizzle with olive oil, then season with salt and pepper.
5. Bake for 20 to 25 minutes, or until the eggplant is golden brown.
6. Spread marinara sauce over each eggplant slice and top with shredded mozzarella and grated Parmesan cheese.
7. Bake for a further 10-15 minutes, or until the cheese melts and bubbles.

Stuffed bell peppers with quinoa and black beans

Ingredients:
- Bell peppers.
- Cooked Quinoa
- Black beans drained and washed.
- Corn kernels
- Diced tomatoes.
- Onions, diced
- Garlic, minced Cumin
- Chili Powder
- Shredded cheese (optional).

Instructions:
1. Preheat the oven to 375° Fahrenheit (190° Celsius).
2. Cut the tops of bell peppers and remove the seeds.

3. In a pan, cook diced onion and garlic until softened.
4. Stir in the cooked quinoa, black beans, corn kernels, chopped tomatoes, cumin, and chili powder.
5. Stuff the bell peppers with the quinoa-black bean mixture.
6. Sprinkle with shredded cheese if desired.
7. Bake for 25–30 minutes, or until the peppers are soft.

Lemon Garlic Shrimp Pasta

Ingredients:
- Peeled and deveined shrimp Linguine pasta.
- garlic, minced
- Olive oil
- Lemon juice
- Chopped fresh parsley and grated Parmesan cheese.
- Salt and pepper.

Instructions:

1. Cook the linguine pasta according to the package instructions.
2. In a medium-size skillet, heat the olive oil.
3. Add the minced garlic and sauté until fragrant.
4. Add the shrimp to the skillet and cook until pink and opaque.
5. Combine cooked pasta, lemon juice, minced parsley, and grated Parmesan cheese.
6. Season with salt and pepper to taste.
7. Serve prawns over lemon garlic pasta.

Vegetable and Tofu Noodle Stir-Fry

Ingredients:

- Cubed tofu.
- Rice noodles
- Mixed vegetables (including broccoli, bell peppers, and snow peas)

- Soy sauce
- Sesame oil
- garlic, minced
- Ginger, grated
- Olive oil

Instructions:

1. Cook the rice noodles according to the package instructions.
2. Heat the olive oil in a big skillet or wok over high heat.
3. Add the cubed tofu and heat until golden brown.
4. Stir in the minced garlic and grated ginger.
5. Stir-fry the mixed vegetables in the skillet until they are soft and crispy.
6. Mix cooked rice noodles with the tofu and veggie mixture.
7. Toss with soy sauce and sesame oil until well combined.

Baked Chicken Parmesan

Ingredients:

- Chicken breasts.
- Italian breadcrumbs
- Grated Parmesan cheese.
- Marinara Sauce
- Shredded mozzarella cheese.
- Olive oil
- Salt and pepper.

Instructions:
1. Preheat the oven to 375° Fahrenheit (190° Celsius).
2. Season the chicken breasts with salt and pepper.
3. Dip the chicken breasts in beaten egg, then coat with a mixture of Italian breadcrumbs and grated parmesan cheese.

4. Place the breaded chicken breasts on a parchment-lined baking sheet.
5. Drizzle with olive oil and bake for 25-30 minutes, or until the chicken is tender.
6. Spread marinara sauce on each chicken breast and top with shredded mozzarella cheese.
7. Bake for a further 10-15 minutes, or until the cheese melts and bubbles.

Vegetarian Spinach and Mushroom Lasagna

Ingredients:
- lasagna noodles.
- Spinach leaves
- Sliced mushrooms and ricotta cheese
- Marinara Sauce
- Shredded mozzarella cheese.
- Grated Parmesan cheese.
- Olive oil and minced garlic.

- Salt and pepper.

Instructions:

1. Preheat the oven to 375° Fahrenheit (190° Celsius).
2. Cook the lasagna noodles according to the package instructions.
3. In a medium-size skillet, heat the olive oil.
4. Sauté sliced mushrooms and minced garlic until they are soft.
5. In a bowl, combine ricotta cheese, cooked spinach leaves, and sautéed mushrooms.
6. Spread marinara sauce on the bottom of a baking dish.
7. Layer the cooked lasagna noodles, ricotta mixture, and shredded mozzarella cheese.
8. Repeat layers until all ingredients have been used, finishing with a layer of marinara sauce and shredded mozzarella.
9. Sprinkle with grated Parmesan cheese.

10. Cover with foil and bake for 30 minutes. Remove the foil and bake for another 15 minutes, or until the cheese is bubbling and golden brown.

Vegetable and Lentil Curry

Ingredients:
- Cooked lentils.
- Mixed vegetables (including carrots, potatoes, and peas)
- Onions, diced
- garlic, minced
- Ginger, grated
- Curry Powder
- Coconut milk
- Vegetable broth with olive oil.
- Salt and pepper.

Instructions:

1. In a large pot, heat the olive oil over medium heat.
2. Sauté the diced onion, minced garlic, and grated ginger until softened.
3. Cook the mixed vegetables until they are slightly soft.
4. Stir in the cooked lentils, curry powder, coconut milk, and vegetable broth.
5. Simmer for 20-25 minutes, or until the veggies are tender and the curry thickens.
6. Season with salt and pepper to taste.

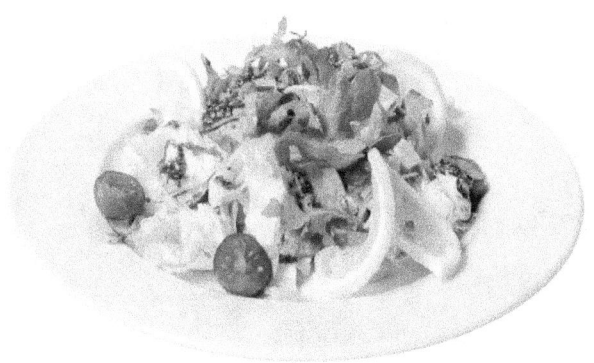

CHAPTER 6: SNACK AND SIDE DISH RECIPES

Greek Yogurt and Mixed Berries

Ingredients:
- Greek yogurt
- Mixed berries (blueberries, strawberries, and raspberries)
- Honey (Optional)
- Instructions:
- Put Greek yogurt in a bowl.
- Garnish with mixed berries.
- Drizzle with honey if preferred.

Cottage Cheese and Pineapple Skewers

Ingredients:
- Cottage Cheese
- Fresh pineapple chunks.

- Skewers

Instructions:
- Thread cottage cheese and pineapple slices onto skewers.
- Serve immediately as a refreshing snack.

Hummus and Vegetable Platter

Ingredients:
- Hummus.
- Mixed vegetables (carrot sticks, cucumber slices, and bell pepper strips)
- Arrange hummus and vegetables on a dish.
- Serve as a healthful, crispy snack.

Trail mix with nuts and seeds

Ingredients:
- Almonds.
- Walnuts

- Pumpkin seeds.
- Sunflower seeds
- Dried cranberries

Instructions:

Combine almonds, walnuts, pumpkin seeds, sunflower seeds, and dried cranberries in a bowl. Divide into snack-sized portions for an easy on-the-go choice.

Whole Grain Crackers with Avocado Mash

Ingredients:
- whole grain crackers.
- Ripe avocado
- Lemon juice
- Salt and pepper.
- Directions: Mash ripe avocado with lemon juice, salt, and pepper.

- Spread avocado mash on whole grain crackers for a tasty snack.
- Side Dishes:

Steamed broccoli with garlic butter

Ingredients:
1. broccoli florets
2. Ingredients: butter and minced garlic.
3. Salt and pepper.
4. Instructions:
5. Steam broccoli florets till soft and crisp.
6. In a small skillet, heat the butter and sauté the minced garlic until fragrant.
7. Drizzle garlic butter over steamed broccoli and season with salt and pepper.

Quinoa Salad With Cranberries and Almonds

Ingredients:

- Cooked Quinoa.
- Dried cranberries
- Sliced almonds
- Fresh parsley, chopped.
- Lemon vinaigrette dressing.

Instructions:

1. In a mixing bowl, add cooked quinoa, dried cranberries, sliced almonds, and chopped parsley.
2. Toss the salad with the lemon vinaigrette dressing.

Roasted Brussels sprouts with Balsamic Glaze

Ingredients:
- half Brussels sprouts and olive oil.
- Balsamic glaze
- Salt and pepper.

Instructions:
1. Preheat the oven to 400° F (200° C).
2. Toss the halved Brussels sprouts with olive oil, salt, and pepper.
3. Roast in the oven for 20-25 minutes, until caramelized and tender.
4. Drizzle with balsamic glaze before serving.

Caprese Salad Skewers

Ingredients:
- Cherry tomatoes
- Fresh mozzarella balls.
- Basil leaves.
- Balsamic glaze
- Skewers

Instructions:
- Thread cherry tomatoes, mozzarella balls, and basil leaves onto skewers.

- Drizzle with balsamic glaze before serving.

Sweet Potato Fries

Ingredients:
- Cut sweet potatoes into fries.
- Olive oil Paprika
- Garlic powder
- Salt and pepper.

Instructions:
1. Preheat the oven to 425° Fahrenheit (220° Celsius).
2. Combine sweet potato fries with olive oil, paprika, garlic powder, salt, and pepper.
3. Spread the fries in a single layer on a parchment-lined baking sheet.
4. Bake for 25-30 minutes, or until crispy. Flip halfway through.

Mango salsa

Ingredients:

- Diced mango,
- red bell pepper,
- red onion, and minced jalapeño pepper (optional).
- Chop fresh cilantro and mix with lime juice.
- Salt and pepper.

Instructions:

1. Dice mango, red bell pepper, red onion, jalapeño pepper (if using), and cilantro.
2. Drizzle with lime juice, then season with salt and pepper.
3. Stir to blend and chill until ready to serve.

Zucchini Noodles With Pesto

Ingredients:

- Zucchini spiralized into noodles.

- Pesto Sauce
- Halve cherry tomatoes and add pine nuts (optional).

Instructions:

- Use a spiralizer to make zucchini noodles.
- Toss the zucchini noodles in pesto sauce until evenly coated.
- If desired, top with halved cherry tomatoes and pine nuts.

Cucumber and Tomato Salad

Ingredients:

- sliced cucumber, halved cherry tomatoes, thinly sliced red onion,
- chopped fresh dill, and Greek yogurt dressing.

Instructions:

- In a mixing bowl, combine sliced cucumber, halved cherry tomatoes, thinly sliced red onion, and chopped fresh dill.
- Toss with Greek yogurt dressing to coat.

Edamame Hummus

Ingredients:
- Edamame (shelled) Tahini
- Lemon juice
- Garlic minced with olive oil.
- Salt and pepper.

Instructions:
1. In a food processor, combine the shelled edamame, tahini, lemon juice, garlic, olive oil, salt, and pepper until smooth.
2. Season to taste, then serve with whole grain crackers or vegetable sticks.

Stuffed bell peppers with quinoa and vegetables

Ingredients:

- Bell peppers.
- Cooked Quinoa
- Mixed vegetables (including maize, peas, and carrots)
- Dice the onion and mince the garlic.
- Tomato sauce
- Italian seasoning.
- Shredded cheese (optional).

Instructions:

1. Preheat the oven to 375° Fahrenheit (190° Celsius).
2. Cut the tops of bell peppers and remove the seeds.
3. In a pan, cook diced onion and garlic until softened.

4. Stir in the cooked quinoa, mixed vegetables, tomato sauce, and Italian seasoning.
5. Stuff the bell peppers with the quinoa and vegetable combination.
6. Sprinkle with shredded cheese if desired.
7. Bake for 25–30 minutes, or until the peppers are soft.

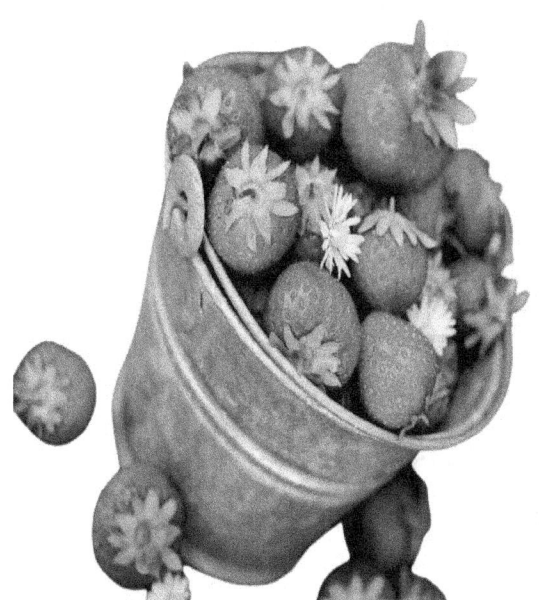

CHAPTER 7: DESSERTS AND SWEET TREATS

Greek yogurt parfait with fresh fruit

Ingredients:

- Greek Yogurt.
- Mixed berries (blueberries, strawberries, and raspberries)
- Honey (Optional)
- Granola (Optional)

Instructions:

1. Layer Greek yogurt, mixed berries, and honey in a glass.
2. Repeat layers until the glass is full.
3. Top with granola if desired.

Baked apples with cinnamon

Ingredients:

- apples.
- Cinnamon and honey (optional)
- Chopped nuts (optional).

Instructions:

1. Preheat the oven to 375° Fahrenheit (190° Celsius).
2. Core the apples and put them in a baking dish.
3. Sprinkle cinnamon on the apples and sprinkle with honey if preferred.
4. Bake for 25 to 30 minutes, or until the apples are soft.
5. Serve warm, with the option of topping with chopped nuts.

Dark chocolate-dipped strawberries

Ingredients:
1. fresh strawberries.
2. Dark chocolate chips.
3. Wash and dry the strawberries completely.
4. Melt dark chocolate chips in a microwave-safe basin, stirring every 30 seconds, until smooth.
5. Dip each strawberry in melted chocolate, coating it about halfway.
6. Place the coated strawberries on a parchment-lined baking sheet.
7. Allow chocolate to set at room temperature, or refrigerate until hard.

Frozen Banana Pops

Ingredients:
- ripe bananas.
- Dark chocolate.

- Optional: chopped nuts or shredded coconut.
- Popsicle sticks

Instructions:
1. Peel and cut bananas in half crosswise.
2. Place a popsicle stick into each banana half.
3. Place the bananas on a parchment-lined baking sheet and freeze until hard.
4. Melt the dark chocolate in a microwave-safe bowl.
5. Dip frozen banana halves into the melted chocolate and top with chopped almonds or shredded coconut, if preferred.
6. Return to the freezer until the chocolate has hardened.

Chia Seed Pudding

Ingredients:
- chia seeds.
- Almond milk (or any milk of your choosing).

- Honey or maple syrup?
- Vanilla extract.
- Fresh fruit for topping.

Instructions:

1. In a bowl, combine the chia seeds, almond milk, honey or maple syrup, and vanilla extract.
2. Stir thoroughly and chill for at least 2 hours or overnight, stirring occasionally to avoid clumping.
3. Serve chilled and topped with fresh fruit.

Frozen Yogurt Bark

Ingredients:

1. Greek Yogurt.
2. Honey or maple syrup?
3. Instructions: Mix berries (blueberries, strawberries, raspberries).
4. Line a baking sheet with parchment paper.

5. In a bowl, combine Greek yogurt and honey or maple syrup.
6. Spread the yogurt mixture evenly over the parchment paper.
7. Sprinkle mixed berries over the yogurt.
8. Freeze for 2–3 hours, or until firm.
9. Divide the frozen yogurt bark into pieces and serve immediately.

Baked peaches with cinnamon and honey

Ingredients:
- Peaches, halved and pitted
- Cinnamon Honey
- Chopped nuts (optional).

Instructions:
1. Preheat the oven to 375° Fahrenheit (190° Celsius).
2. Place the peach halves cut side up in a baking tray.

3. Sprinkle cinnamon over the peaches, then sprinkle with honey.
4. Bake for 20–25 minutes, or until the peaches are soft.
5. Serve warm, with the option of topping with chopped nuts.

Coconut Date Balls

Ingredients:

- Pitted Medjool dates
- Unsweetened, shredded coconut
- Almond flour
- Vanilla extract.

Instructions:

1. In a food processor, combine pitted dates, shredded coconut, almond flour, and vanilla essence until the mixture holds together.
2. Roll the mixture into little balls with your hands.

3. Optional: Coat the balls with additional shredded coconut.
4. Refrigerate for a minimum of 30 minutes before serving.

Homemade Fruit Sorbet

Ingredients:
- Mixed frozen fruits (e.g., berries, mango, pineapple).
- Honey or maple syrup is optional.
- Lemon juice

Instructions:
1. In a blender or food processor, combine the frozen fruit, honey or maple syrup (if using), and lemon juice.
2. Blend until smooth and creamy, adding a little water if needed to aid in blending.

3. Serve immediately as soft-serve, or transfer to a container and freeze for a firmer consistency.

Pumpkin Oatmeal Cookies

Ingredients:
- rolled oats.
- Pumpkin puree
- Maple syrup
- Cinnamon Nutmeg
- Chopped walnuts or raisins are optional.

Instructions:
1. Preheat the oven to 350°F/175°C and line a baking sheet with parchment paper.
2. In a mixing bowl, combine rolled oats, pumpkin puree, maple syrup, cinnamon, nutmeg, and chopped walnuts or raisins, if preferred.

3. Scoop spoonfuls of the mixture onto the prepared baking sheet and gently flatten with a fork.
4. Bake for 12-15 minutes, or until the cookies are golden brown on the edges.
5. Allow the cookies to cool before serving.

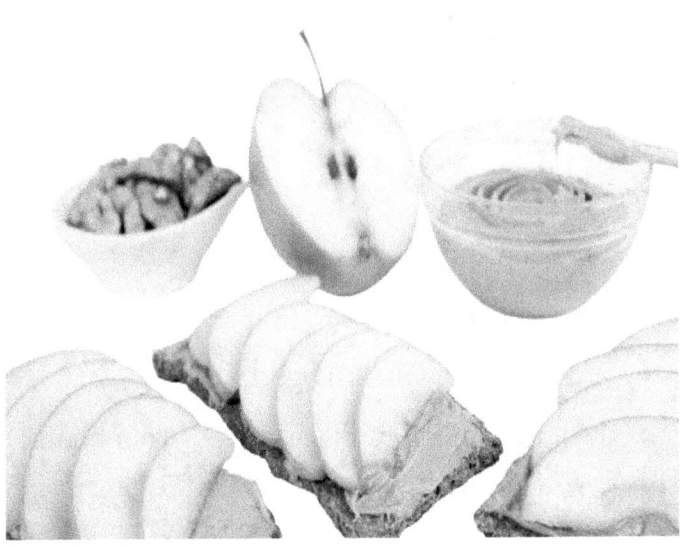

CHAPTER 8 : BEVERAGES

Calcium-Rich Smoothie

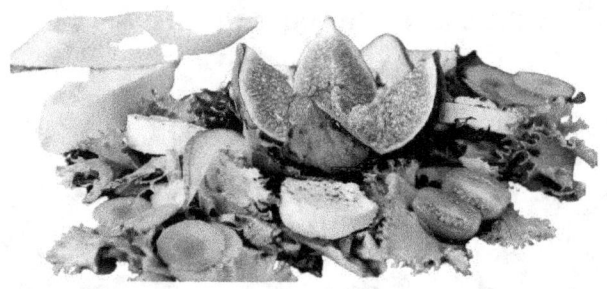

Ingredients:

- One cup spinach.
- One ripe banana.
- 1/2 cup plain Greek yogurt.
- 1/2 cup almond milk (or milk of your choice)
- 1 tablespoon almond butter.
- 1/2 teaspoon of vanilla extract.
- Add honey or maple syrup to taste.

Instructions:

1. Combine all of the ingredients in a blender.
2. Blend until smooth and creamy.
3. Pour into a glass and drink immediately.

Almond Milk

Ingredients:

- 1 cup raw almonds (soaked overnight)
- 4 cups of water.
- Add honey or maple syrup to taste.
- 1/2 teaspoon of vanilla extract (optional)

Instructions:

1. Rinse soaked almonds and discard the soaking water.
2. Blend almonds and water in a high-speed blender until smooth.
3. Using a nut milk bag or cheesecloth, strain the mixture into a big bowl.
4. If desired, stir in honey or maple syrup as well as vanilla essence.

5. Keep almond milk in the refrigerator for up to 3-4 days.

Green Tea

Ingredients:
1. Green tea bags or loose tea leaves.
2. Hot water
3. Honey or lemon slices are optional.
4. Instructions:
5. Steep green tea bags or loose leaves in boiling water for 3 to 5 minutes.
6. Remove tea bags or sieve the tea leaves.
7. Sweeten with honey or lemon slices, if preferred.
8. Serve hot or chill in the refrigerator to make iced green tea.

Bone-building Berry Smoothie

Ingredients:

- 1/2 cup frozen mixed berries.
- 1/2 ripe banana.
- 1/2 cup plain Greek yogurt.
- 1/2 cup almond milk (or milk of your choice)
- 1 tablespoon of chia seeds.
- One teaspoon of honey or maple syrup (optional)

Instructions:
1. Combine all of the ingredients in a blender.
2. Blend until smooth and creamy.
3. Pour into a glass and drink immediately.

Calcium-boosting Orange Smoothie

Ingredients:
- One orange, peeled and segmented
- 1/2 cup plain Greek yogurt.
- 1/2 cup almond milk (or milk of your choice)
- 1 tablespoon honey or maple syrup.
- Ice cubes

Instructions:

1. Combine orange segments, Greek yogurt, almond milk, honey or maple syrup, and ice cubes in a blender.
2. Blend until smooth and creamy.
3. Pour into a glass and serve immediately.

Strawberry Kiwi Calcium Smoothie

Ingredients:
- 1/2 cup frozen strawberries.
- One kiwi, peeled and sliced
- 1/2 cup plain Greek yogurt.
- 1/2 cup almond milk (or milk of your choice)
- 1 tablespoon honey or maple syrup.

Instructions:

1. Combine frozen strawberries, sliced kiwi, Greek yogurt, almond milk, and honey or maple syrup in a blender.

2. Blend until smooth and creamy.
3. Pour into a glass and drink immediately.

Homemade Cashew Milk

Ingredients:
- Soak 1 cup raw cashews overnight.
- 4 cups of water.
- Add honey or maple syrup to taste.
- 1/2 teaspoon of vanilla extract (optional)

Instructions:
1. Rinse cashews and discard the soaking water.
2. Blend cashews and water in a high-speed blender until smooth.
3. Using a nut milk bag or cheesecloth, strain the mixture into a big bowl.
4. If desired, stir in honey or maple syrup as well as vanilla essence.
5. Refrigerate cashew milk for up to 3-4 days.

Banana-Almond Smoothie

Ingredients:

- One ripe banana.
- 1 tablespoon almond butter.
- 1/2 cup almond milk (or milk of your choice)
- 1/2 cup plain Greek yogurt.
- 1 tablespoon honey or maple syrup.
- Ice cubes

Instructions:

1. Blend ripe bananas, almond butter, almond milk, Greek yogurt, honey or maple syrup, and ice cubes in a blender.
2. Blend until smooth and creamy.
3. Pour into a glass and serve immediately.

Vanilla almond milk

Ingredients:

- One cup blanched and peeled almonds.

- 4 cups water and 1 tablespoon honey or maple syrup.

Instructions:
1. 1 teaspoon vanilla extract.
2. In a blender, combine the almonds and water until smooth.
3. Using a nut milk bag or cheesecloth, strain the mixture into a big bowl.
4. Return the strained milk to the blender, then add honey or maple syrup and vanilla extract.
5. Blend until thoroughly blended.
6. Refrigerate for up to three or four days.

Chocolate almond milk

Ingredients:
- Soak 1/2 cup almonds overnight.
- 2 glasses of water.
- 2 tablespoons of unsweetened cocoa powder.
- Two teaspoons of honey or maple syrup

- 1/2 teaspoon of vanilla extract.

Instructions:
1. Rinse soaked almonds and discard the soaking water.
2. In a blender, combine almonds, water, cocoa powder, honey or maple syrup, and vanilla extract until smooth.
3. Using a nut milk bag or cheesecloth, strain the mixture into a big bowl.
4. Serve chilled over ice, or warm gently over the stove.

Golden milk (turmeric latte)

Ingredients:
- 1 cup almond milk (or other milk of choice).
- 1 teaspoon ground turmeric.
- Half a teaspoon of crushed cinnamon
- 1/4 teaspoon of ground ginger.
- 1 tablespoon honey or maple syrup.

- A pinch of black pepper.

Instructions:
1. In a small saucepan, heat the almond milk over medium heat.
2. Whisk in the ground turmeric, cinnamon, ginger, honey or maple syrup, and a pinch of black pepper.
3. Heat till heated, but not boiling.
4. Pour into a mug and enjoy.

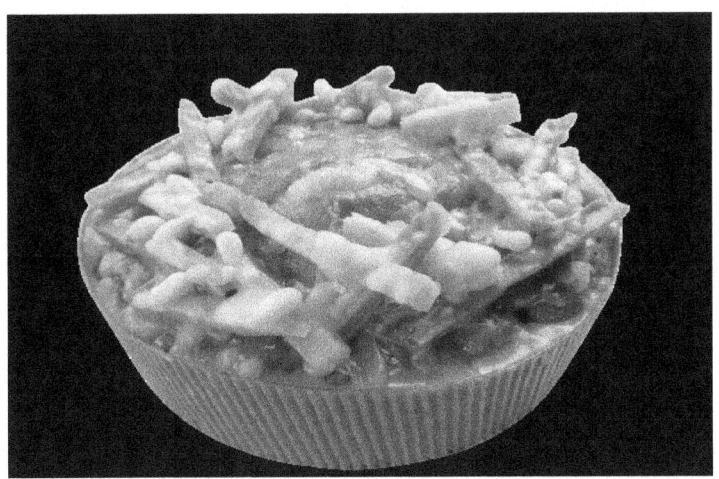

CHAPTER 9: BONUSES
7-DAY MEAL PLANNING

Day 1

Breakfast: Calcium-Rich Smoothie (spinach, banana, Greek yogurt, almond milk, almond butter, honey.

Lunch: Quinoa salad with cranberries and almonds.

Snack: Greek Yogurt and Mixed Berries

Dinner: Baked salmon with steamed broccoli and brown rice.

Day 2:

Breakfast: Green Tea, Whole Grain Toast, and Avocado Mash

Lunch: lentil soup with a side of whole grain bread.

Snack: Cottage cheese and pineapple skewers.

Dinner: Vegetable and Tofu Noodle Stir-Fry.

Day 3:

Breakfast: Bone-Building Berry Smoothie (berries, banana, Greek yogurt, almond milk, and chia seeds)

Lunch: Spinach salad with grilled chicken, cherry tomatoes, and balsamic vinaigrette.

Snack: Trail mix with nuts and seeds.

Dinner: Stuffed bell peppers with quinoa and vegetables.

Day 4:

Breakfast: Almond Milk Oatmeal with sliced banana and chopped walnuts.

Lunch: Caprese Salad Skewers with Whole Grain Crackers

Snack: Homemade Fruit Sorbet.

Dinner: Lemon Garlic Shrimp Pasta and Steamed Asparagus

Day 5:

Breakfast: Greek yogurt parfait with fresh fruits and granola.

Lunch: Vegetable and lentil curry with brown rice.

Snack: Dark chocolate-dipped strawberries.

Dinner: Baked Chicken Parmesan with Roasted Brussels sprouts.

Day 6:

Breakfast: Coconut Date Balls with a Cup of Green Tea

Lunch: Zucchini Noodles with Pesto, with a side of cucumber and tomato salad

Snack: Frozen Yogurt Fruit Popsicles (with Greek yogurt and mixed berries).

Day 7:

Breakfast: pumpkin oatmeal cookies and a glass of homemade cashew milk.

Lunch: Edamame Hummus, Whole Grain Pita Bread, with Sliced Bell Peppers

Snack: baked apples with cinnamon and a drizzle of honey.

Dinner: Sweet potato fries with mango salsa.

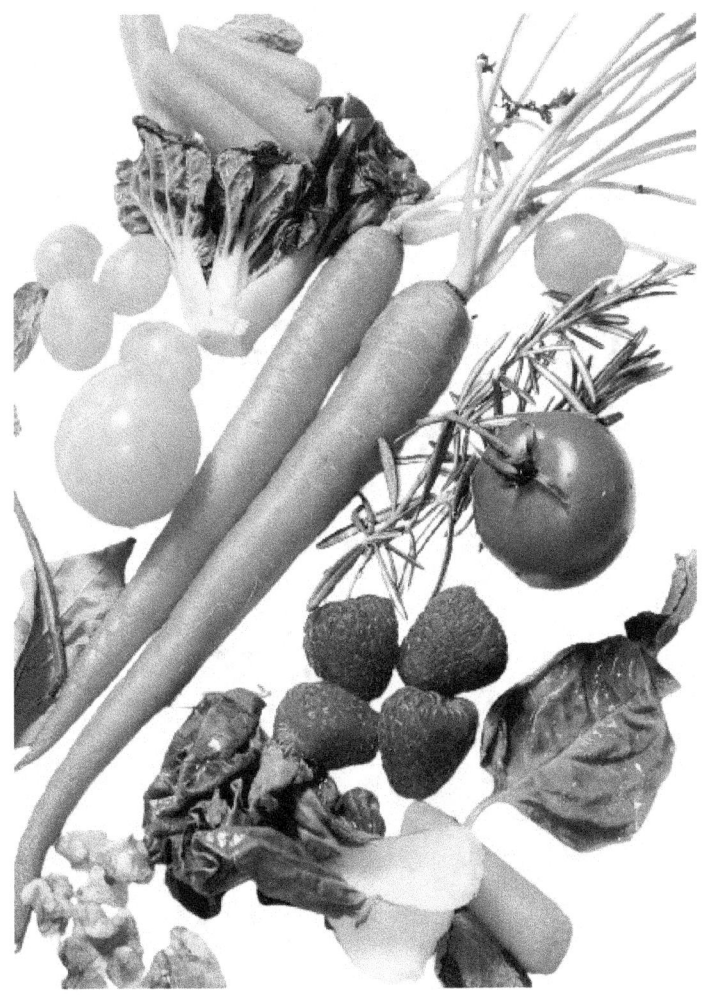

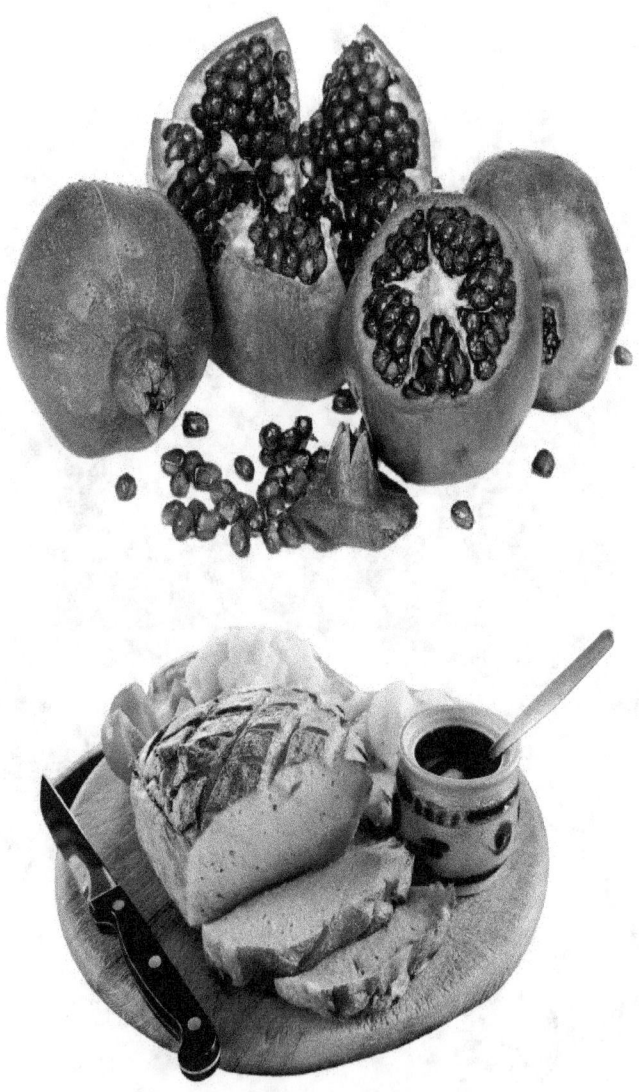

CONCLUSION

Additional materials

Additional resources for anyone seeking more information and support on osteoporosis, including the Osteoporosis Diet Cookbook:

Online Support Communities:
Joining osteoporosis-specific online forums and support groups can provide helpful insights, tips, and encouragement from others going through similar experiences. Websites such as Osteoporosis.org and HealthUnlocked provide supportive forums where you can connect with others suffering similar issues.

Books and publications:
Explore other books and publications on osteoporosis and nutrition to have a better grasp of

the condition and its dietary therapy. Look for credible books written by healthcare professionals or registered dietitians who specialize in bone health.

Consultation with Health Professionals:
Schedule an appointment with your healthcare practitioner, a registered dietitian, or a nutritionist to discuss your particular dietary requirements and receive specialized recommendations based on your health state and goals.

Educational Workshops & Seminars:
Attend instructional courses, seminars, or webinars on osteoporosis and nutrition. These seminars frequently feature expert speakers who provide useful insights and actionable techniques for improving bone health via nutrition and lifestyle.

Nutritional Counseling Services:

Consider receiving nutritional counseling from a licensed dietitian who specializes in osteoporosis management. A competent specialist can help you accomplish your health objectives by providing specific nutritional advice, meal planning assistance, and continuous coaching.

Bone Health Organizations and Foundations:
Investigate resources offered by recognized bone health organizations and foundations, such as the National Osteoporosis Foundation (NOF) and the International Osteoporosis Foundation (IOF). These organizations provide a plethora of information, instructional tools, and support services to people living with osteoporosis.

Cooking Classes & Workshops:
Enroll in cooking seminars or workshops geared toward making nutritional and bone-healthy meals. Many culinary schools, community centers, and

health groups teach workshops about the necessity of including calcium-rich foods, vitamin D sources, and other bone-building minerals into your diet.

Podcasts and webinars:
Listen to podcasts or watch webinars that cover osteoporosis, nutrition, and healthy living. These media platforms frequently contain interviews with experts in the industry, who provide vital insights and practical advice for improving bone health through food and lifestyle changes.

Research studies and clinical trials:
Stay up to date on current research studies and clinical trials looking at novel advances in osteoporosis treatment, such as dietary interventions and nutritional supplements. Participation in research projects may provide possibilities to advance scientific understanding while also gaining access to cutting-edge treatments or interventions.

Education Websites & Online Resources:

Research reliable websites and internet resources for osteoporosis education and awareness. Websites such as Mayo Clinic, Harvard Health Publishing, and WebMD provide detailed articles, fact sheets, and resources on osteoporosis diagnosis, treatment, and prevention.

By using these extra materials in conjunction with the Osteoporosis Diet Cookbook, people can develop a better understanding of osteoporosis care and empower themselves to make informed decisions about their bone health and overall well-being.

www.ingramcontent.com/pod-product-compliance
Lightning Source LLC
Chambersburg PA
CBHW071101240526
45471CB00016B/2298